75 E-JUICE RECIPES & COOKBOOK 2.0

Shane H. Alexander

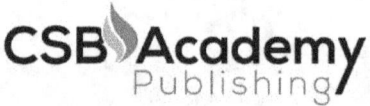

CSB Academy Publishing Company.
P. O. Box 966
Semmes, Alabama 36575, USA

Design and Layout
By
Angie Anderson
First Edition

CONTENT AT A GLANCE

INTRODUCTION

In my last book e-juice recipe and cookbook, I concentrated more on the "cooking "part and less on the recipe side, so I have decided to do the 2.0 of the book where I mention more recipe and less on cooking. But you don't have to read the first one to enjoy this one. Both are stand alone and pretty easy to follow.

But I would like to mention once again that I am not really a writer I never was, just wanted to share the knowledge I gathered so my sincere apology in advance in case you find errors in this book. Some of the ingredients may be hard to understand at first, but the chances are that wherever you buy your e-liquid supplies from will carry them, best is do a Google search for the best suppliers as they change so fast and often. But I did include a few reputable ones on here, and no I don't have any affiliate association with them, so feel free to shop around for the best deal.

If you have been vaping for a while like me, then I bet that you're craving some new flavors and rightly so! Buying the same cheap flavors can start to kill the joy of smoking and some of those high-end eLiquids may just be out of your financial reach right now, not to mention that when you purchase eJuices from the market or online on a frequent basis, it can become really expensive to sustain your hobby.

Well, if you are among the many people facing the disappointment that follows after vaping the same flavors of eLiquids or if it has lost its effect on you and you want to try something new, then here's a book that can help you! If you are an avid vaper, you must know that you can make your own eJuice as well but there's a bit of a problem with that, you don't have the best eJuice recipes!

Preparing your perfect eJuice recipe and getting all the ingredients in the right quantity is quite a bit of work. It requires patience and constant trial and error to reach the goal, and until you're done perfecting one recipe, you may be exhausted, and unwilling try further. Experimenting with making your own eJuice can thus, result in a tenuous experiment that drains your energy in the end and leaves you shoving it aside, only to find yourself saving and spending money on pre-made eJuices that you are bound to buy.

But wait, things don't have to be that bad, and you don't have to exhaust yourself trying to perfect your eJuice recipes. I have gone through the trouble for you because I was keen to learn and perfect my art of eJuices for myself and my friends, and I'm ready to share it here with you!

After spending hours, days, and months I have perfected some great tasting super yummy eJuice recipes that you all will love to try as well. I am sure of it because my friends already can't get enough of them.

Whether or not you are an avid e-cigarette smoker, this book right here is for you!

It is no longer a problem for you to make your own eJuice and it no longer remains a problem to try new flavors. This short and super easy recipe book rids you of all your problems of preparing eJuices and gives you a new flavor to make for each day. You will have no trouble following the instructions as everything is laid down in an easy to follow step by step guide and the recipes have been perfected to get the best flavor. All you need to do is follow the instructions and viola!

You have a new eJuice flavor to try!

So just when you have been hooked onto the relatively new trend of e-cigarettes and are in the phase of life where you are ready to experiment with different flavors, you can simply pick up this book and start following the simple recipe instructions it gives to prepare yourself a new and different flavor.

WHAT DOES THIS BOOK INCLUDE?

This book covers the basics of preparing eJuices by yourself as well as the ingredients that are required in detail, as those who are new to it can find it difficult to adjust to the terms and ingredients as they are a bit different from conventional cigarette ingredients.

In my last book as Is aid I talked more about the process and less about the actual recipes, but one thing is worth mentioning that in that book I did lay out a process of extracting the nicotine from tobacco leaf, which has become a very popular hobby for a lot of vapers, so if you are interested in learning how to do that, check out that book.

Once you understand the basics of the ingredients, we will cover the equipment required, which isn't much. It is easy, and you can do it with a bit of effort.

Next up, once you are ready, you can get started with the recipes where I bring tried and tested eJuice recipes to you that are sure to elevate your e-cigarette experience. There isn't one or two, but five different categories of eJuice recipe flavors that I have covered in this book. You will find it interesting to explore recipes in the following flavor categories:

- Fruit Flavored
- Drink Flavored
- Minty Madness
- Sweet Punch
- Dessert

Now I'm sure you're excited to get your hands on your eJuice in these exciting recipe flavor categories, so without further ado, let's get started.

GETTING STARTED: WHAT YOU'LL NEED

Vaping is as much about great taste choices as it is about individuality and I understand that, as with everything else in life that quickly loses its charm, your once favorite eJuices may have too!

We're getting to the recipes but before we nose dive into them, let me touch upon the main ingredients and the equipment you will need to prepare your recipe. I want you to understand that perfecting and crafting a new flavor of eJuices is an art, and that takes time. Understanding what a recipe is made of will better equip you with the knowledge and understanding of the recipe itself.

With practice, you may even start to understand how you can alter the ingredients' ratio to create a mild or stronger flavor and all that will come when you understand the dynamics of the underlying ingredients.

INGREDIENTS

Any eJuice recipe contains three main ingredients which include nicotine, PG or VG and the flavors itself. Getting the right ratio or mix of the ingredients is very important in creating a new flavor but I have accomplished that feat for you. Let's have a quick look at the ingredients:

PG OR VG

Propylene glycol or vegetable glycerin, commonly referred to as PG or VG, is a diluent for the nicotine and flavors that are highly concentrated. It dilutes them to create a pleasurable flavor. The PG or VG makes up most of the formula as it's the base or carrier fluid in the recipe. You must know that PG gives a stronger throat hit when you vape, and VG is used to create more vapor.

PG and VG are both slightly different in their taste, viscosities, and throat feet and most eJuices contain a mix of both to create the right feel. Some common ratios that both these ingredients are used in are 70/30, 30/70 and 50/50. Flavored eJuices are usually diluted using PG but using a ratio of both is the recommended way to create the right vapor.

FLAVORS

The most important part of the recipe is the flavor; given that you're looking for a bit of taste in your eJuice. However, let me tell you that you can make your eJuice without flavor as well. That is referred to as "neat" eLiquid and isn't a common vapor choice. You can easily purchase your flavor anywhere that sells e-cigarettes and its accompanying products, and it shouldn't be a problem to find it online as well.

NICOTINE

Nicotine has its own flavor, and it is one of the main and most important ingredients in an e-cigarette acting as a stimulant for the eJuice. It tastes different at different strengths, but since it's a potent chemical, it is best advised that you use it carefully and limit its addition to the recipe to less than 36 mg. Even that could be too much, but anything above that could be downright fatal.

EQUIPMENT

Making your own eliquid isn't easy, but at the same time, it's exciting. You get to try all new and different kinds of flavors that you concoct in your leisure time, enhancing your e-cigarette experience. However, keep in mind that some of the ingredients that you are going to be working with are dangerous and require a certain level of diligence and care when using them, such as nicotine, so it's essential to be prepared with the right equipment before you start trying different recipes out.

Here is the equipment you will need to prepare your eJuice recipe:

Gloves

The first and foremost important thing is to have a pair of gloves at your disposal. Nicotine is dangerous to work with as it can be absorbed into your skin upon contact. Always wear a pair of gloves before starting to make your recipe.

Syringes

After gloves, the second most important thing is syringes and pipettes because you need something to accurately transfer the right quantities of liquid from your supply of the different ingredients into your eJuice recipe creation. Using syringes, you can transfer the exact amount of nicotine, PG/VG or flavor that the recipe demands and transfer it to the container in which you are preparing it. It will also allow you to be in control of the quantities of your new flavor in case you want to replicate it. You will know exactly how much of each ingredient to use to get the exact same flavor again.

Bottles

Since you're experimenting, you will need some bottles to prepare and store your eJuice. For the purpose, buy plastic drip tip bottles as these are also cost effective. You can also re-use these bottles when making different flavors. The advantage of using smaller bottles while you're experimenting with recipes is that you are able to do your math and measurements as precisely as possible. The quantities you work with when making your eJuice are already small, making it harder to measure in large containers.

MAKING YOUR ELIQUID

Before I give you the recipes, I have gone through immense trouble perfecting for your benefit. I'll walk you through the process of preparing it from scratch, in case if you are entirely new to it. I understand it could get really costly to purchase the premade eJuice once the flavors start getting limited. However, once you learn the process, you can start your experimenting with my recipes and try new and exciting flavors for your eJuice.

One important aspect of preparing the eJuice recipe is to be able to reproduce it later. It can get really difficult to get that perfect flavor that will soothe your taste buds and tastes good in your mouth as the smoke hits your throat. Unless you are very experienced, it can take a long time for you to reach the perfect recipe for a certain flavor and not to mention, discover a whole lot of others. I have gone through the pains of all this experimentation for you and noted down precise measurements and careful notes for all the perfectly flavored recipes that taste good. Now all you need to do is learn how to make the recipe and get started with the recipes mentioned in this eBook.

STEPS TO PREPARE YOUR RECIPE

Step 1: Determine Nicotine Strength

The first thing that you need to do is determine the strength of nicotine in the eJuice and how much will be needed for that. Getting the wrong nicotine strength and volume can lead to an unpleasant experience. Here's a quick guide on how you can alter and determine the nicotine strength in the various recipes and suit it to your taste. Although each recipe listed mentions the right volume of nicotine to use, once you know how it is measured, you can calculate your own nicotine strength based on your preference.

Determine the amount of nicotine required in milligrams:

(Strength in mg/ml) *(volume in ml) = amount of nicotine in mg

For example, if you want to make 50 ml of 8mg/ml liquid, so you will need 50*8= 400mg of nicotine for your 50 ml formula.

Now, to calculate the volume to use:

(Amount needed)/strength of diluted nicotine) = volume to use

Continuing with the same example:

If you have 100 mg/ml, diluted nicotine, you will need:

400mg/ (100mg/ml) = 4 ml

Step 2: Transfer of Nicotine

Now this is where your syringe and drip tip bottle will come in use. You will use it to the transfer the nicotine. Don't forget to wear your gloves while doing so. Moving on with the same example; if you're making 8 mg/ml with 25 mg/ml PG nicotine, you will need a clean syringe to extract 16 ml nicotine from the container.

It can be tricky to draw the exact amount of nicotine. The easiest way to do is to draw a little more than you need and carefully depress the plunger to the required mark, in this case, its 16-ml. Make sure to keep the syringe pointed into the bottle while depressing so that there is no wastage of the diluted nicotine, minimizing chances of error as well.

Another thing to look out for, are any air bubbles in the syringe which can affect your measurements. If you notice any air bubbles in the syringe, it is important to tap it to bring the air to the top and depress the plunger carefully to get rid of it. Just try and bring the liquid to the tip of the needle to get rid of air bubbles.

Step 3: Add Flavor

Once you have successfully transferred the right amount of nicotine in the bottle, you next have to add the flavor. Keep in mind that the recommended dilution for flavors is 10%, but you can change it according to your taste and how light or heavy you want to keep the flavor. Again, the recipes provide you a perfect blend of all the exactly measured ingredients, but you can alter it according to your taste.

The flavor will have to be transferred to the bottle using a syringe in the same way that you transferred the nicotine. So, for example, if you are making 50 ml of the eJuice, you will need 5 ml of the flavor according to the recommended 10 % dilution level.

Another important thing to take note of here is that flavor concentrates are complicated artificial flavors and adding more flavor doesn't necessarily mean you will make your recipe better. You may want to increase the flavor in your eJuice, and that's okay, but over flavoring it can lead to washing the flavor out and leaving it tasting more like it is the chemical constituents that make up the flavor. Also, the flavors you use tend to affect the dilution level as some flavors are stronger than others at the same level of dilution.

As a good rule of thumb, you should keep the entire volume of flavors you are using between 10 and 15 percent of the total volume of the eLiquid you are preparing. It also helps to check the package instructions from the manufacturer where you get your flavor from to have an idea of the required percentage.

Mixing different flavors become more complex but don't worry; you will find a variety of recipes in this eBook to suit your taste and preferences.

Step #4- Add the Base or Diluents to Complete Liquid

In this example, you will find that there already is a lot of PG from the nicotine and flavoring in the eJuice recipe so as a diluent you can use VG. To make your 50 ml of eLiquid, you have already included 16 ml of nicotine and 5 ml of flavoring. That leaves us with 29 ml of room to add the base to reach that amount of eLiquid. Again, you can use a clean syringe to transfer the VG to the bottle.

At this point, you should be using carefully marked bottles to know how much volume they contain because when you add the base, you don't want to miss it from the required and suggested measurement. Bottles may also differ in size, which can overthrow you off the entire process of mixing the right quantities. Before starting, know how much liquid your bottle can hold and mark your required volume levels so that there's no confusion.

If you want to use a specific blend of PG/VG in your recipe, you can do it using some quick math. To make a 50/50 blend of PG/VG, you will require 4 ml more of PG and 25 ml more of VG in this example. To make a higher blend, you will have to use a higher strength of the diluted nicotine, which reduces the total amount of PG.

Step #5- Shake It Up

Congratulations! Now you have every ingredient that is required to make the eJuice, and all you need to do is cap the bottle and shake it up. Make sure you to tightly secure the cap so that there is no chance of a leakage. Shake the bottle for several minutes at least so that the nicotine and flavor thoroughly mix together.

Remember that the ingredients may separate over time, so you may have to thoroughly shake it before each vape.

One quick thing to mention here is that when you store your eJuice, you may notice the flavor changing over time. This is known as steeping and is a result of chemical reactions taking place between the oxygen in the air and the ingredients. So keep in mind that time also plays an important role in flavoring and helps blend it better. Some eJuices tend to taste better after left to age for a few days or a week.

When you shake the recipe for use, open the cap, and let the formula sit for a few days to get the ideal combination and right mix. Some flavors such as vanillas, creams, and custards, enhance through steeping and stand out quite a bit if left for a few days.

With this basic process of preparing an eJuice recipe at your disposal now, I hope you are ready to start trying the recipes I have perfected for you. Happy vaping!

One more thing I want to mention before we dive deep into the recipes, you will notice a few name of ingredients that may be hard to find, but if you do a Google search, you will find them as I found them from various eLiquid supply stores online.

Here is a list of a few I bought from, but not as not every one of them gave me a good experience, so I will leave it up to you to decide and do your own search and decide where you should buy from. Just remember not all supply stores are created equal.

http://www.ecigexpress.com/diy-e-liquid.html

https://www.mtbakervapor.com/electronic-cigarette-diy-supplies/

http://diye-liquidsupplies.com/

http://www.myfreedomsmokes.com/mixing-supplies.html

Here is a link to a list someone put up on the e-cig forum

https://www.e-cigarette-forum.com/forum/threads/diy-vendor-supplies-list.133074/

RECIPES

FRUIT FLAVORED

1. Strawberry and Peach Delight

Makes 30 ml

Ingredients	ml	Grams
PG dilutant	4.2	4.36
VG dilutant	23.1	29.13
Nicotine juice 100 mg	0.9	1.13
Juicy Peach	0.9	0.9
Strawberry	0.9	0.9

PG/VG ratio: 20/80

2. Berries and Cream

Makes 10 ml

Ingredients	ml	Grams
PG dilutant	0.2	0.21
VG dilutant	4.0	5.08
Strawberry PA	0.8	0.87
Bavarian cream PA	0.7	0.55
Blueberry PA	0.7	0.76
Ethyl Maltol	0.1	0.11
DDL	0.2	0.22
Base nicotine liquid	3.5	3.71

PG		

PG/VG ratio: 60/40

3. Smoked Apple

Makes 10 ml

Ingredients	*ml*	*Grams*
PG dilutant	0.9	0.95
VG dilutant	4.0	5.08
PA Apple	0.5	0.55
DV Virginia	1.0	1.09
MTS Vape Wizard	0.1	0.11
Base nicotine liquid PG	3.5	3.71

PG/VG: 60/40

4. Kiwi Strawberry

Makes 20 ml

Ingredients	*ml*	*Grams*
PG dilutant	0.9	0.95
VG dilutant	4.0	5.08
PA Apple	0.5	0.55
DV Virginia	1.0	1.09
MTS Vape Wizard	0.1	0.11
Base nicotine liquid PG	3.5	3.71

PG/VG ratio: 60/40

5. Kiwi Strawberry Punch

Makes 20 ml

Ingredients	ml	Grams
PG dilutant	2.6	2.7
VG dilutant	13.4	16.9
Nicotine juice 100 mg (100% VG)	0.6	0.76
Strawberry	1.6	1.6
Kiwi	0.8	0.8
DX Sweet Cream	0.4	0.4
Toasted Marshmallow	0.6	0.6

PG/VG ratio: 30/70

6. Fruity Custard

Makes 10 ml

Ingredients	ml	Grams
PG dilutant	0.45	0.47
VG dilutant	5.95	7.51
Nicotine juice 100 mg (100% PG)	0.6	0.62
Marshmallow	0.2	0.2
Sweetener	0.1	0.1
Blueberry	0.5	0.49
Milk chocolate	0.2	0.2
Sweet cream	0.5	0.49
Vanilla custard	1	1

PG/VG ratio: 30/70

7. Banana Delight

Makes 30 ml

Ingredients	ml	Grams
PG dilutant	2.7	2.8
VG dilutant	20.4	25.73
Nicotine juice 100 mg (100% PG)	0.6	0.76
Bananas foster	1.5	1.5
Cotton candy loran	0.9	0.9
Bavarian cream	0.6	0.6
Vanilla bean IC	2.4	2.4
Sweet cream	0.9	0.9

PG/VG ratio: 30/7

8. Iced Watermelon

Makes 10 ml

Ingredients	ml	Grams
PG dilutant	0.5	0.53
VG dilutant	4.0	5.08
TFA watermelon	0.8	0.87
Inawera menthol	0.2	0.22
Kandi-hed aniseed	0.6	0.65
Kandi-hed eucalyptus	0.2	0.22
Base nicotine liquid PG	0.2	3.71
Inawera	0.2	0.9

pitaya/dragon fruit		

PG/VG ratio: 40/60

9. Blueberry

Makes 10 ml

Ingredients	ml	Grams
PG dilutant	2.0	0.53
VG dilutant	7.1	5.08
Base nicotine liquid (PG)	3.5	3.71
Blueberry	2.0	2.18

PG/VG ratio: 40/60

10. Cherry Cascade

Makes 20 ml

Ingredients	ml	Grams
PG dilutant	2.0	2012
VG dilutant	7.1	9.02
Base nicotine liquid (VG)	6.9	8.76
Ethyl Maltol	0.4	0.44
Cherry cascade TW	3.6	3.92

PG/VG ratio: 30/70

11. Pineapple and strawberry

Makes 10 ml

Ingredients	ml	Grams
PG dilutant	0.5	0.53
VG dilutant	4.0	5.08
Base nicotine liquid (PG)	3.5	3.71
Peach juicy	0.6	0.65
Ripe strawberry	1.0	1.09
Pineapple	0.4	0.44

PG/VG ratio: 60/40

12. Grapefruit Madness

Makes 20 ml

Ingredients	ml	Grams
PG dilutant	1.3	1.38
VG dilutant	10.0	12.7
Base nicotine liquid (PG)	6.9	7.31
Grapefruit inawera	1.0	1.09
Red power flavor	0.2	0.22
Grenadine flavor	1.0	0.65

PG/VG ratio: 50/50

13. Lychee

Makes 10 ml

Ingredients	ml	Grams
PG dilutant	1.2	1.27
VG dilutant	4.0	5.08
Base nicotine liquid (PG)	3.5	3.71
Grenadine flavor X	0.4	0.44

Lychee	0.6	0.65
Cactus (Inawera)	0.3	0.33

PG/VG ratio: 60/40

14. Cheesy Blueberry

Makes 30 ml

Ingredients	ml	Grams
PG dilutant	0.15	0.16
VG dilutant	21	26.49
Base nicotine liquid (PG)	3.75	3.89
Blueberry FW	1.5	1.5
Cinnamon Danish Swirl	1.5	1.5
Cheese cake	1.2	1.2
Graham cracker FW	0.9	0.9

PG/VG ratio: 30/70

15. Lemon Explosion

Makes 10 ml

Ingredients	ml	Grams
PG dilutant	0.5	0.53
VG dilutant	4.0	5.08
Base nicotine liquid (PG)	3.5	3.71
Lime zinger	0.8	0.87
Sherbet lemon	1.2	1.31

PG/VG ratio: 60/40

16. Black Ice

Makes 10 ml

Ingredients	ml	Grams
PG dilutant	1.4	1.48
VG dilutant	4.0	5.08
Base nicotine liquid (PG)	3.5	3.71
Flavor art menthol	0.5	0.55
TFA's blackcurrant	0.6	0.65

PG/VG ratio: 60/40

17. Strawberry Watermelon

Makes 30 ml

Ingredients	ml	Grams
VG dilutant	21.2	26.74
Base nicotine liquid (VG)	2.5	3.15
Milk	0.75	0.75
Watermelon TFA	0.75	0.75
Bubble gum	0.75	0.75
Blueberry cotton candy FW	0.75	0.75
Strawberry	1.5	1.5
Strawberry (ripe)	1.5	1.5
Sour (TPA)	0.3	0.3

PG/VG ratio: 21/79

18. Kiwi Strawberry

Makes 15 ml

Ingredients	ml	Grams
PG dilutant	1.95	2.03
VG dilutant	10.5	13.25
Base nicotine liquid (PG)	0.45	0.47
Kiwi double TPA	0.6	0.6
Sweet strawberry	1.2	1.2
Marshmallow	0.3	0.3

PG/VG ratio: 30/70

19. Strawberry and Banana

Makes 100 ml

Ingredients	ml	Grams
VG dilutant	87	109.71
Base nicotine liquid (PG)	0	0
Banana cream (LA)	6	6
Strawberry (LA)	5	5
Vanilla crème	2	2

PG/ VG ratio: 13/87

20. Strawberry Éclair

Makes 20 ml

Ingredients	ml	Grams
PG dilutant	1.7	1.77
VG dilutant	14	17.66
Base nicotine liquid (PG)	0.8	0.83
Bavarian cream (TPA)	0.6	0.6
Cake (yellow) (FW)	0.3	0.3
Biscuit (INAWERA)	0.4	0.4
Strawberry ripe (TPA)	0.8	0.8
Cheesecake (Graham Crust) (TPA)	0.3	0.3
Sugar cookie (CAP)	0.4	0.4
Strawberry (TPA)	0.3	0.3
Vanilla swirl (TPA)	0.4	0.4

PG/VG ratio: 30/70

DRINK FLAVORED

1. Citrus Refresher

Makes 10 ml

Ingredients	ml	Grams
PG dilutant	1.	1.17
VG dilutant	4.0	5.08
Base nicotine liquid (PG)	3.5	3.71
Inawera lemon	0.3	0.33
Inawera lime ball	0.3	0.33
Capella sweet tangerine	0.3	0.33
TW gold standard ice menthol	0.5	0.55

PG/VG ratio: 60/40

2. Citrab Delight

Makes 20 ml

Ingredients	ml	Grams
PG dilutant	2.6	2.76
VG dilutant	8.0	10.16
Base nicotine liquid (PG)	6.9	7.31
LT lemon mix	0.2	0.22
DV Absinthe	2.0	2.18
LT Orange	0.1	0.11
Inawera Lime	0.1	0.11
Ethyl maltol	0.1	0.11

PG/VG ratio: 60/40

3. Black Cherry and Absinthe Drink

Makes 20 ml

Ingredients	ml	Grams
PG dilutant	0.2	0.21
VG dilutant	10.0	12.7
Base nicotine liquid (PG)	6.9	7.31
Absinthe	1.4	1.53
Black cherry	0.8	0.87
Koolada	0.2	0.22
Sweet strawberry	0.4	0.44
Ethyl maltol	0.1	0.11

PG/VG ratio: 50/50

4. Winter jack

Makes 10 ml

Ingredients	ml	Grams
PG dilutant	0.5	0.53
VG dilutant	4.0	5.08
Base nicotine liquid (PG)	3.5	3.71
FA Kentucky bourbon	1.0	1.09
FW apple jax	1.0	1.09

PG/VG ratio: 60/40

5. Frosted Roll

Makes 14 ml

Ingredients	ml	Grams
VG dilutant	10.78	0.53
Base nicotine liquid (VG)	0.42	0.53
Cinnamon dash	1.26	1.26

Capella super sweet	0.14	0.14
Graham crust	0.42	0.42
Frosted donut (TPA)	0.28	0.28
Pie crust (TPA)	0.14	0.14
Vanilla cupcake (TPA)	0.56	0.56

PG/VG ratio: 20/80

6. Cherry Cola Mix

Makes 10 ml

Ingredients	ml	Grams
PG dilutant	1.0	1.06
VG dilutant	4.0	5.08
Base nicotine liquid (PG)	3.5	3.71
Cola (inawera concentrate in drops)	1.0	1.09
Cherry (Inawera concentrate in drops)	0.5	0.55

PG/VG ratio: 60/40

7. Blackcurrent and Grape Mix

Makes 10 ml

Ingredients	ml	Grams
PG dilutant	0.1	0.11
VG dilutant	4.0	5.08
Base nicotine liquid (PG)	3.5	3.71
Blackcurrent (inawera concentrate in drops)	1.2	1.31
Raspberry (inawera concentrate in drops	0.8	0.87
Grape (inawera concentrate in drops)	0.4	0.44

PG/VG ratio: 60/40

8. Fruit Mix

Makes 10 ml

Ingredients	ml	Grams
PG dilutant	0.5	0.53
VG dilutant	4.0	5.08
Base nicotine liquid (PG)	3.5	3.71
Apple (Inawera concentrate in drops	1.0	1.09
Pear (Inawera concentrate in drops)	0.6	0.65
Plum (inawera concentrate in drops)	0.4	0.44

PG/VG ratio: 60/40

9. Honey and Lime Mix

Makes 7 ml

Ingredients	ml	Grams
VG dilutant	5.59	7.05
Base nicotine liquid (VG)	0.58	0.73
Banana	0.04	0.04
Cranberry	0.07	0.07
Blood orange (FW)	0.04	0.04
Italian lemon sicily (CAP)	0.12	0.12
Honey (Inawera)	0.02	0.02
Lime	0.02	0.02
Milkstone	0.2	0.2
Papaya	0.02	0.02
MTS vape wizard	0.01	0.01
Papaya (TPA)	0.02	0.02
Pink guava	0.04	0.04
Raspberry	0.09	0.09
Wild melon	0.16	0.16

PG/VG ratio: 12/88

10. Honeydew and Cream

Makes 60 ml

Ingredients	ml	Grams
VG dilutant	21	26.49
Base nicotine liquid (PG)	30	31.08
Honeydew (TPA)	6	6
Sweet cream (TFA)	3	3

PG/VG ratio: 65/35

11. Grape Drink

Makes 10 ml

Ingredients	ml	Grams
PG dilutant	0.5	0.53
VG dilutant	4.0	5.08
Base nicotine liquid (PG)	3.5	3.71
TPA grape candy	1.0	1.09
(KH) skittles	1.0	1.09

PG/VG ratio: 60/40

12. Cherry Pomegranate

Makes 30 ml

Ingredients	ml	Grams
PG dilutant	3.2	3.32
VG dilutant	21	26.49
Base nicotine liquid (PG)	1.8	1.86
Acai berry	1.5	1.5
Pomegranate deluxe	1.5	1.5

(TPA)		
Tutti frutti	1	1

PG/VG ratio: 30/70

13. Lime Cola

Makes 25.01 ml

Ingredients	ml	Grams
PG dilutant	4.82	5
VG dilutant	13.44	16.95
Base nicotine liquid (50/50 VG/PG)	3.13	3.59
Ina cactus	0.06	0.06
TFA cola	0.5	0.5
TFA green apple	1	1
TFA key lime	0.25	0.25
TFA lemon	0.75	0.75
TFA raspberry	0.75	0.75
TFA sweetener	0.31	0.31

PG/VG ratio: 40/60

14. Irish Mocha

Makes 30 ml

Ingredients	ml	Grams
PG dilutant	4.05	4.2
VG dilutant	21	26.49
Base nicotine liquid (PG)	3.6	3.73
Caramel (FA)	0.15	0.15
Chocolate overload	0.15	0.15
EM	0.15	0.15
Irish cream (FA)	0.45	0.45
Tiramisu (FA)	0.15	0.15
Vienna cream (FA)	0.3	0.3

PG/VG ratio: 30/70

15. Caramel Coffee

Makes 10 ml

Ingredients	ml	Grams
PG dilutant	1.7	1.80
VG dilutant	4.0	5.08
Base nicotine liquid (PG)	3.5	3.71
Flavor art espresso crème	0.5	0.55
TFA DX Caramel original	0.3	0.33

PG/VG ratio: 60/40

16. Peanut Butter

Makes 30 ml

Ingredients	ml	Grams
VG dilutant	23.4	29.51
Base nicotine liquid (PG)	1.8	1.86
Chocolate loran oils	1.8	1.8
Peanut butter-vaping zone	1.8	1.8
Graham cracker TPA	0.6	0.6
Whipped cream	0.6	0.6

PG/VG ratio: 22/78

17. Splenda

Ingredients	ml	Grams
VG dilutant	24.24	30.57
Base nicotine liquid (VG)	0.9	1.13
Cinnamon roll	3	3
Ethyl maltol	0.3	0.3
Vanilla cupcake	0.6	0.6
Sugar cookie	0.96	0.96

PG/VG ratio: 16/84

18. Comfy Lemon

Makes 30 ml

Ingredients	ml	Grams
VG dilutant	24.6	31.03
Base nicotine liquid (PG)	1.8	2.27
Bourbon FA	0.3	0.3
Coconut FA	0.15	0.15
Condensed milk FA	0.3	0.3
Joy FA	0.6	0.6
Cookie FA	0.9	0.9
Meringue FA	0.6	0.6
Torrone FA	0.15	0.15
Lemon sicily FA	0.3	0.3
Yogurt FA	0.3	0.3

PG/VG ratio: 12/88

19. Sweet Tobacco

Makes 30 ml

Ingredients	ml	Grams
PG dilutant	6.96	7.22
VG dilutant	15.24	19.22
Base nicotine liquid (30/70 VG/PG)	1.8	2.15
TPA sweet cream	0.6	0.6
Biscuit FA	0.9	0.9
Cheesecake TPA	0.9	0.9
Cowboy Blend	1.5	1.5
Maxx blend	1.5	1.5
Vanilla custard	0.6	0.6

PG/VG ratio: 45/55

20.Strawberry Milkshake

Makes 30 ml

Ingredients	ml	Grams
VG dilutant	24.6	31.03
Base nicotine liquid (PG)	1.8	1.86
Malted milk TPA	1.2	1.2
Strawberry ripe TPA	1.8	1.8
Vanilla bean IC TPA	0.6	0.6

PG/VG Ratio: 18/82

1. Peppermint Delight

Makes 10 ml

Ingredients	ml	Grams
PG dilutant	0.7	0.74
VG dilutant	4.0	5.08
Base nicotine liquid (PG)	3.5	3.71
DV Absinthe	1.5	1.64
TPA sweetener	0.2	0.22
TPA Peppermint	0.1	0.11

PG/VG ratio: 60/40

2. Extreme Mint

Makes 10 ml

Ingredients	ml	Grams
PG dilutant	0.5	0.53
VG dilutant	4.0	5.08
Inawera eucalyptus with mint	0.2	3.71
Flavor west- yum berry	0.9	0.22
Flavor West- razzleberry	0.9	0.98
Flavor west- cherry berry	0.1	0.11

PG/VG ratio: 60/40

3. Heavenly Delight

Makes 20 ml

Ingredients	ml	Grams
PG dilutant	1.6	1.70
VG dilutant	8.0	10.16
Base nicotine liquid (PG)	6.9	7.31
TPA bittersweet chocolate	1.4	1.53
TPA sweet cream	1.0	1.09
TPA Peppermint	0.8	0.87
TPA French vanilla	0.2	0.22
TPA ethyl maltol	0.1	0.11

PG/VG ratio: 60/40

4. Holey Mint

Makes 10 ml

Ingredients	ml	Grams
PG dilutant	1.1	1.17
VG dilutant	4.0	5.08
Base nicotine liquid (PG)	3.5	3.71
TPA peppermint	1.0	1.09
Menthol	0.2	0.22
Koolada	0.1	0.11
Ethyl maltol	0.2	0.22

PG/VG ratio: 60/40

5. Fisherman's Friend Delight

Makes 10 ml

Ingredients	ml	Grams
PG dilutant	0.3	0.32
VG dilutant	4.0	5.08
Base nicotine liquid	3.5	3.71

(PG)		
Inawera anise	0.3	0.33
Inawera licorice	0.6	0.65
Perfumers apprentice peppermint	0.2	0.22
Perfumers apprentice koolada	0.2	0.22
Decadent vapours mentholyptus	0.7	0.76
Menthol crystals mix	0.2	0.22

PG/VG ratio: 60/40

6. <u>Minty menthol</u>

Makes 10 ml

Ingredients	ml	Grams
PG dilutant	0.7	0.74
VG dilutant	4.0	5.08
Base nicotine liquid (PG)	3.5	3.71
Peppermint	1.0	1.09
Menthol	0.1	0.11
Aniseed	0.2	0.22
Bavarian cream	0.5	0.55

PG/ VG ratio: 60/40

7. <u>Mint Candy</u>

Makes 20 ml

Ingredients	ml	Grams
PG dilutant	2.3	2.44
VG dilutant	8.0	10.16
Base nicotine liquid (PG)	6.9	7.31
Hangsen mint candy	2.0	2.18
Ethyl maltol	0.2	0.22
Menthol	0.6	0.65

PG/VG ratio: 60/40

8. Berry Mint

Makes 10 ml

Ingredients	ml	Grams
PG dilutant	0.5	0.53
VG dilutant	4.0	5.08
Base nicotine liquid (PG)	3.5	3.71
Cherry berry	0.5	0.55
Menthol	1.5	1.64

PG/VG ratio: 60/40

9. Mint Candy Extreme

Makes 10 ml

Ingredients	ml	Grams
PG dilutant	2.78	2.89
VG dilutant	5	6.31
Base nicotine liquid (PG)	0.42	0.44
Blue Raspberry cotton candy CAP	1	1
Cool mint	0.4	0.4
Two apples	0.4	0.4

PG/VG ratio: 50/50

10. Radioactive

Makes 15 ml

Ingredients	ml	Grams
PG dilutant	2.25	2.34

VG dilutant	8.62	10.87
Base nicotine liquid (VG)	1.88	2.37
Absinthe	0.3	0.3
Quince	1.95	1.95

PG/VG ratio: 30/70

1. Vanilla Butter

Makes 10 ml

Ingredients	ml	Grams
PG dilutant	1.6	1.70
VG dilutant	4.0	5.08
Base nicotine liquid (PG)	3.5	3.71
Vanilla custard	0.6	0.65
Butter	0.2	0.22
Peppermint	0.1	0.11

PG/VG: 60/40

2. Sweet And Sour Balls

Makes 10 ml

Ingredients	ml	Grams
PG dilutant	0.9	0.95
VG dilutant	4.0	5.08
Base nicotine liquid (PG)	3.5	3.71
Inawera blueberry	0.5	0.55
Inawera lime	0.1	0.11
Inawera blackcurrant	0.6	0.65
Inawera peer	0.1	0.11
Loran raspberry	0.1	0.11
Ethyl maltol	0.1	0.11
Wera garden Bahraini Apple Gold	0.1	0.11

PG/VG: 60/40

3. Sweet Chocolate

Makes 20 ml

Ingredients	ml	Grams
PG dilutant	6.2	6.57
VG dilutant	3.1	3.94
Base nicotine liquid (VG)	6.9	8.76
Vanilla	1.2	1.31
Hazelnut (roasted)	1.2	1.31
Sweetener	0.2	0.22
Double dark chocolate	1.2	1.31

PG/VG: 50/50

4. Citrus Absinthe

Makes 10 ml

Ingredients	ml	Grams
PG dilutant	0.4	0.42
VG dilutant	3.0	3.81
Base nicotine liquid (PG)	3.5	3.71
Absinthe DV	1.4	1.53
Green apple (capella)	0.6	0.65
Citrus mix (FA)	0.5	0.55
Licorice FA	0.2	0.22
Lemon sickly	0.1	0.11

PG/VG: 70/30

5. Coconut Delight

Makes 10 ml

Ingredients	ml	Grams
PG dilutant	1.2	1.27
VG dilutant	4.0	5.08

	ml	Grams
Base nicotine liquid (PG)	3.5	3.71
Hangsen RY4 concentrate	1.0	1.09
Flavourart hazelnut	0.1	0.11
Inawera coconut	0.2	0.22

PG/VG dilutant: 60/40

6. Sour Mix

Makes 10 ml

Ingredients	ml	Grams
PG dilutant	0.5	0.53
VG dilutant	4.0	5.08
Base nicotine liquid (PG)	3.5	3.71
Swedish fish-falvourwest	0.5	0.55
Cherry-flavourart	0.3	0.76
Blue raspberry- the rebranded range	0.5	0.55
Strawberry-flavourart	0.3	0.33

PG/VG: 60/40

7. Milky Chocolate Coconut

Makes 10 ml

Ingredients	ml	Grams
PG dilutant	1.8	1.91
VG dilutant	3.0	3.81
Base nicotine liquid (PG)	3.5	3.71
HiLIQ dark chocolate	0.7	1.09
TPA Dulce De Leche	0.0	0.00

PG/VG ratio: 70/30

8. Blackcurrant With A Twist

Makes 10 ml

Ingredients	ml	Grams
PG dilutant	0.7	0.74
VG dilutant	4.0	5.08
Base nicotine liquid (PG)	3.5	3.71
Capella anise	0.3	0.33
Inawera blackcurrant	1.0	1.09
Decadent absinthe	0.3	0.33
Flavor west blackjack	0.2	0.22

PG/VG: 60/40

9. Strawberry Bubblegum Delight

Makes 20 ml

Ingredients	ml	Grams
PG dilutant	2.5	2.65
VG dilutant	8.0	10.16
Base nicotine liquid (PG)	6.9	7.31
Strawberry juice	1.6	1.74
Bubblegum	1.0	1.09

PG/VG: 60/40

10. Refreshing Berry Punch

Makes 30 ml

Ingredients	ml	Grams
PG dilutant	4.0	4.24
VG dilutant	9.0	11.43
Base nicotine liquid (PG)	10.4	11.02
Rainbow sherbert TPA	2.4	2.62
Sour TPA	0.9	0.98
Rainbow drops TPA	1.5	1.64
Harvest berry	0.3	0.33
Raspberry CAP	0.3	0.33
Strawberry	0.3	0.33
Key lime	0.3	0.33
Ethyl maltol	0.3	0.33

PG/VG: 70/30

11. Menthol And Cherry

Makes 10 ml

Ingredients	ml	Grams
PG dilutant	2.0	2.12
VG dilutant	4.0	5.08
Base nicotine liquid (PG)	3.5	3.71
Tino d'milano cherry	0.3	0.33
Menthol crystals	0.2	0.22

PG/VG ratio: 70/30

12. Calipitter Lime

Makes 10 ml

Ingredients	ml	Grams
PG dilutant	0.7	0.74
VG dilutant	4.0	5.08
Base nicotine liquid (PG)	3.5	3.71
Mom & pop's calipitter chow flavour	1.0	1.09
Inawera deluxe tobacco flavor concentrate	0.3	0.33
Perfumer's apprentice key lime flavor	0.5	0.55

PG/VG ratio: 60/40

13. Mint Dark Chocolate

Makes 20 ml

Ingredients	ml	Grams
PG dilutant	1.1	1.17
VG dilutant	8.0	10.16
Base nicotine liquid (PG)	6.9	7.31
Bittersweet chocolate	2.0	2.18
Crème de menthe	2.0	2.18

PG/VG ratio: 60/40

14. Hot Cinnamon Delight

Makes 10 ml

Ingredients	ml	Grams
PG dilutant	0.5	0.53
VG dilutant	4.0	5.08

Base nicotine liquid (PG)	3.5	3.71
Flavor West cinnamon red hot	0.8	0.87
TPA Jamaican Rum	0.3	0.33
Flavor West cinnamon hot tamale	0.8	0.87
TPA clove	0.2	0.22

PG/VG ratio: 60/40

15. Coconut ice

Makes 10 ml

Ingredients	ml	Grams
PG dilutant	0.5	0.53
VG dilutant	4.0	5.08
Base nicotine liquid (PG)	3.5	3.71
Koolada	0.5	0.55
Capella coconut	1.5	1.64

PG/VG ratio: 60/40

1. Vanilla Fudge

Makes 10 ml

Ingredients	ml	Grams
PG dilutant	0.8	0.85
VG dilutant	4.0	5.08
Base nicotine liquid (PG)	3.5	3.71
Blackcurrent	0.4	0.44
Vanilla fudge	1.0	1.09
Aniseed	0.2	0.22
Dulce de leche	0.1	0.11

PG/VG ratio: 60/40

2. Banana Custard

Makes 20 ml

Ingredients	ml	Grams
PG dilutant	4.1	4.35
VG dilutant	6.0	7.62
Base nicotine liquid (PG)	6.9	7.31
Banana	1.0	1.09
Van custard	1.2	1.31
Bavarian cream	0.6	0.65
Dulce de leche	6.9	0.22

PG/VG ratio: 70/30

3. Nutmeg Custard

Makes 10 ml

Ingredients	ml	Grams
PG dilutant	1.5	1.59
VG dilutant	3.0	3.81
Base nicotine liquid (PG)	3.5	3.71
Dulche de leche	0.2	0.22
Cap van custard	1.3	1.42
Nutmeg	0.2	0.22
Bavarian cream	0.3	0.33

PG/VG ratio: 70/30

4. Cherry Pie

Makes 20 ml

Ingredients	ml	Grams
PG dilutant	1.1	1.17
VG dilutant	8.0	10.16
Base nicotine liquid (PG)	6.9	7.31
Capella pie crust	0.6	0.65
Capella black cherry	3.4	3.71

PG/VG ratio: 60/40

5. Banana Bread

Makes 10 ml

Ingredients	ml	Grams
PG dilutant	1.7	1.8
VG dilutant	4.0	5.08
Base nicotine liquid (PG)	3.5	3.71
Strawberry	0.1	0.11

TPA banana nutbread	0.5	0.55
Banana	0.1	0.11
Strawberry	0.1	0.11

PG/VG ratio: 60/40

6. <u>Butterscotch Dessert</u>

Makes 20 ml

Ingredients	*ml*	*Grams*
PG dilutant	0.9	0.95
VG dilutant	8.0	10.16
Base nicotine liquid (PG)	6.9	7.31
Butterscotch	0.4	0.44
Bavarian cream	1.2	1.31
Sweetener	0.2	0.22
Vanilla custard	2.4	2.62

PG/VG ratio: 60/40

7. <u>Vanilla Cream Surprise</u>

Makes 10 ml

Ingredients	*ml*	*Grams*
PG dilutant	0.6	0.64
VG dilutant	4.0	5.08
Base nicotine liquid (PG)	3.5	3.71
Apple pie	0.8	0.87
Vienna cream	0.8	0.87
Sweetener	0.1	0.11
Cocoa	0.2	0.22
MTS Vape wizard	0.1	0.11

PG/VG ratio: 60/40

8. <u>Citrus Cake</u>

Makes 10 ml

Ingredients	ml	Grams
PG dilutant	0.0	0.00
VG dilutant	3.0	3.81
Base nicotine liquid (PG)	3.5	3.71
Lemon and lime	0.4	0.44
New York cheesecake	0.6	0.65
Vanilla custard	1.0	1.09
Natural vanilla	1.0	1.09
Sour flavor	0.5	0.55

PG/VG ratio: 70/30

9. <u>Chocolate Custard</u>

Makes 10 ml

Ingredients	ml	Grams
PG dilutant	0.5	0.53
VG dilutant	4.0	5.08
Base nicotine liquid (PG)	3.5	3.71
Capella vanilla custard	0.5	0.55
Inawera chocolate	0.5	0.55
Perfumer's apprentice almond amaretto	0.5	0.55
Capella graham cracker	0.5	0.55

PG/VG ratio: 60/40

10. Apple cinnamon

Makes 20 ml

Ingredients	ml	Grams
PG dilutant	2.5	2.65
VG dilutant	8.0	10.16
Base nicotine liquid (PG)	6.9	7.31
Capella apple pie	1.6	1.74
Capella cinnamon Danish swirl	1.0	1.09

PG/VG ratio: 60/40

CONCLUSION

So there you go. Now, you have a wide variety of flavors at your disposal that are going to enhance your vaping experience. With these well researched and perfected recipes at hand, you no longer have to buy costly eJuice for yourself. Simply select a recipe that suits your taste from these choices available to you, create it, and have fun!

I hope you have as much fun vaping these different flavors as I have had while perfecting them! In the meanwhile, make sure you follow all the directions given in the book correctly and vigilantly.

Use the right equipment and be very careful while handling the ingredients.

Safety comes first, so follow the directions and enjoy the large variety of eJuice recipe flavors listed here.

If you like my work, and think I have provided some value here, please give me a review on this book, it will make my world little brighter and I do want to thank you from bottom of my heart for you buying my book.

Happy vaping folks! Enjoy!

www.ingramcontent.com/pod-product-compliance
Lightning Source LLC
Chambersburg PA
CBHW071257280526
45788CB00004B/1739